Best Foreplay Tips and Techniques for Romantic Couples

20+ Top Foreplay Tips and Ideas for Better Sex Tonight plus Tips You'll Be Dying to Try

Cheryl Bach

Best Foreplay Tips and Techniques for Romantic Couples

Publisher: IntimateInk Press

Email: intimateinkpress@gmail.com

This book is a work of nonfiction intended for informational purposes only. The content of this book is based on the author's research, knowledge, and experience, and it is provided with the understanding that the author and publisher are not engaged in rendering legal, medical, or professional advice. The information in this book is not a substitute for professional guidance or assistance. Readers should consult with relevant professionals for advice and assistance regarding their specific situations. The author and publisher disclaim any liability for any loss or risk, personal or otherwise, which is incurred as a consequence, directly or indirectly, of the use and application of any of the contents of this book.

Cover design by IntimateInk Press

Interior layout and design by IntimateInk Press

Printed in USA

Fonts: Google fonts

Image: Freepik.com. This cover has been designed using assets from Freepik.com

First Edition: 2024

Distributed by Amazon.com, Inc.

Cheryl Bach

Table of Contents

Introduction

Foreplay is often an underrated aspect of sexual intimacy. However, it can play a significant role in enhancing sexual pleasure and strengthening emotional bonds between partners. Foreplay involves any non-penetrative sexual activity that occurs before intercourse, including kissing, touching, and oral sex.

Many couples overlook the importance of foreplay in their sexual encounters. But skipping foreplay can lead to a lackluster sexual experience that fails to fully satisfy both partners. Engaging in foreplay can lead to better communication, stronger emotional connections, and ultimately, more satisfying sex.

Benefits of Foreplay in a Romantic Relationship

Increases Sexual Arousal: Foreplay helps to increase sexual arousal by stimulating erogenous zones in the body. Kissing, touching, and caressing can help to build anticipation and desire, leading to more intense sexual pleasure.

Helps to Create Emotional Connection: Foreplay can help to build emotional connections between partners. It allows couples to be more attuned to each other's needs, desires, and preferences. This emotional intimacy can enhance trust and strengthen the bond between partners.

Improves Sexual Performance: Engaging in foreplay can help to improve sexual performance by increasing blood flow to the genitals, increasing lubrication, and helping partners to relax and feel more comfortable during sex.

Enhances Orgasms: Foreplay can enhance the intensity and frequency of orgasms for both partners. By taking the time to stimulate erogenous zones and build arousal, both partners are more likely to experience more intense and satisfying orgasms.

Reduces Stress and Anxiety: Foreplay can be an effective way to reduce stress and anxiety in both partners. It helps partners to relax and enjoy the moment, which can have a calming effect on the mind and body. By reducing stress and anxiety, couples are more likely to experience satisfying sex.

Helps to Boost Self-Esteem: Engaging in foreplay can help to boost self-esteem and body confidence in both partners. When couples indulge in sensual activities, they become more aware of their bodies and the pleasure that they can give and receive. This awareness can lead to greater body confidence and self-esteem, which can, in turn, enhance sexual pleasure.

As you can see, foreplay is an essential aspect of sexual intimacy. It not only enhances physical pleasure but also strengthens emotional bonds between partners. By taking the time to engage in foreplay, couples can improve their sexual experiences and build more meaningful relationships.

In this book, we'll explore 20+ top foreplay tips and techniques designed to help couples improve their sexual experiences and enjoy better sex tonight. From exploring erogenous zones to introducing new types of stimulation, we'll guide you through a range of exciting and pleasurable foreplay techniques.

Whether you're a new couple looking to spice up your sex life or a long-term couple looking for new ways to deepen your emotional and physical connection, this book is for you. So, get ready to explore the many benefits of foreplay and discover tips and techniques that will transform your sex life.

11

Understanding Foreplay

Foreplay is any sexual activity that leads up to intercourse. It includes a range of non-penetrative sexual activities such as kissing, touching, oral sex, and erotic massage. By engaging in foreplay activities, couples can build excitement, connection, and arousal before having sex.

Types of Foreplay

There are many different types of foreplay, and couples can experiment with a variety of techniques to find what works best for them.

Some common types of foreplay include:

Kissing: Kissing is one of the most popular forms of foreplay. Kissing stimulates the lips and tongue, which are both erogenous zones.

Touching: Touching involves caressing your partner's body in a sensual way. This can include running your hands over their skin, stroking their hair, or gently gripping their hips.

Oral Sex: Oral sex involves performing sexual activities with the mouth, lips, and tongue. It can be performed on both male and female partners and is a great way to build arousal and intimacy.

Erotic Massage: Erotic massage is a sensual form of touch that involves using your hands to massage your partner's erogenous zones. It can be a relaxing and enjoyable way of building arousal and intimacy.

Role-Playing: Role-playing involves acting out sexual fantasies or scenarios. It can be a fun and exciting way to experiment with fantasies and add a sense of novelty to your sexual encounters.

Importance of Communication before Foreplay

Before engaging in any sexual activity, it is important to communicate with your partner.

Effective communication allows couples to understand each other's needs, boundaries, and desires. This is especially important during foreplay because it involves a lot of physical intimacy and vulnerability. Sharing your thoughts and desires with your partner can help ensure that both partners are comfortable and enjoying themselves.

Before engaging in foreplay, take the time to talk to your partner about what you like and don't like, what turns you on, and what boundaries you have. Communication can also help to build anticipation and tension, leading to more satisfying sexual experiences.

During foreplay, continue to communicate with your partner. Pay attention to their body language and verbal cues, and check in with them to make sure they are comfortable and enjoying themselves. If something doesn't feel good or if you want to try something new, speak up.

Remember, consent is key. Always make sure that both partners are comfortable and consenting to the sexual activities you engage in. Respect your partner's boundaries and avoid pressuring them into anything they're not comfortable with.

Cheryl Bach

In summary, foreplay is a crucial aspect of sexual intimacy that can enhance physical pleasure and strengthen emotional bonds between partners. There are many different types of foreplay, and couples can experiment with a variety of techniques to find what works best for them. However, communication is key before and during foreplay. Being open and honest with your partner can help ensure that both partners are comfortable, enjoying themselves, and having a satisfying sexual experience. So, take the time to explore and experiment with new foreplay techniques, but remember to always prioritize communication and consent.

III

Top 20+ Foreplay Tips and Techniques

Sensual Massages

- Use warm oil and start with gentle caresses, gradually increasing pressure as you go.

- Pay special attention to erogenous zones like the neck, ears, back, and inner thighs.

- Add some variety to your massage technique by using different textures, like a feather or silk scarf.

Erotic Kissing Techniques

- Try kissing your partner's neck while lightly nibbling on their earlobe.

- Alternate between soft, tender kisses and deeper, more passionate ones.

- Experiment with gently biting your partner's lower lip.

Creative Use of Sex Toys

- Use a vibrator to stimulate your partner's clitoris during foreplay.

- Explore your partner's body with a feather tickler or tickling glove.

- Use a blindfold to heighten your partner's senses and anticipation.

Cheryl Bach

Dirty Talk and Role-Playing

- Describe in detail what you would like to do to your partner, or what you want them to do to you.

- Don't be afraid to use vulgar language or to say things that might make you blush.

- Try acting out a scenario like a seductive nurse/patient or teacher/student.

Nipple Play and Breast Massage

- Use varying degrees of pressure and experiment with different techniques like sucking and nibbling.

- Alternate between stimulation of the nipples and kissing the neck or lips.

- Use a feather tickler to gently run over the nipples, enhancing sensitivity and arousal.

Oral Sex Techniques

- Experiment with light touches with your lips and tongue before increasing the pressure and suction.

- Use your hands to explore and massage surrounding areas while providing oral stimulation.

- Use ice cubes or hot tea to provide temperature play sensations during oral sex.

Erotic Fantasies and Storytelling

- Share your deepest desires and fantasies with your partner.

- Set the mood with lighting, music, or props to help act out a fantasy.

- Take turns coming up with short erotic stories or scenarios to create a sexy atmosphere.

Seductive Striptease

- Choose a sexy outfit that your partner will love, and practice your moves in front of the mirror.

- Make use of props like a chair or a feather boa to add a sultry element to your routine.

- Don't be afraid to make eye contact with your partner while performing, and use your body language to tease and tantalize.

Mutual Masturbation

- Take turns pleasing each other while watching and encouraging your partner.

- Use different techniques and speeds to build anticipation and arousal.

- Try incorporating toys like vibrators or dildos into your mutual masturbation sessions for added pleasure.

Bondage and BDSM

- Establish boundaries and a safe word before beginning any bondage or BDSM activities.

- Start with lighter activities like gentle restraint or role-playing before moving on to more intense bondage or domination techniques.

- Use props like blindfolds, handcuffs, or floggers to enhance the experience.

IV

Tips You'll Be Dying to Try

When it comes to foreplay, there are endless possibilities. Couples who are looking to spice things up may want to consider exploring their sexual fantasies, mutual exploration of erogenous zones, incorporating food and drink, sensory deprivation, temperature play, tantric sex techniques, erotic kissing games, sex in public places, and incorporating music and lighting.

Exploring Sexual Fantasies

Exploring your sexual fantasies with your partner can be a great way to spice up your sex life. Talk openly and honestly with your partner about what turns you on. Set clear boundaries and make sure that both partners are comfortable with the situation. Some couples might enjoy role-playing and acting out different scenarios, while others might prefer simply describing their fantasies to each other.

Mutual Exploration of Erogenous Zones

Erogenous zones are areas of the body that are particularly sensitive to sensual touch. While many people may automatically think of the genitals as being the primary erotogenic zone, there are many other areas of the body that can be a source of pleasure and arousal. These may include the neck, ears, inner thighs, nipples, and even the feet. Try slowly exploring each other's bodies, taking note of what feels good and what doesn't. Don't be afraid to experiment with different types of touch and pressure as well.

Incorporating Food and Drink

Incorporating food and drink into your foreplay routine can add an element of playfulness and sensuality. You might try feeding each other fruit or chocolate, or even experiment with some edible body paint or whipping cream. Just be sure to keep things clean and hygienic!

Sensory Deprivation

Sensory deprivation involves restricting one or more senses to heighten the sensation of the others. Blindfolds, earplugs, and even restraints can be used to create an incredibly intimate experience between partners. Try blindfolding your partner and slowly exploring their body with your hands, or using restraints to tease and titillate.

Temperature Play

Temperature play involves using hot and cold sensations to enhance sexual pleasure. You might try incorporating ice cubes, a cold metal spoon, or even a heating pad into your play. As always, make sure to talk to your partner about what they're comfortable with and set boundaries beforehand.

Tantric Sex Techniques

Tantric sex is an ancient practice that aims to cultivate intimacy and connection between partners. Breathing techniques, meditation, and even certain yoga poses can all be used to enhance sexual pleasure and intimacy. Tantric sex takes practice, but the resulting connection and mutual satisfaction can be incredibly rewarding.

Erotic Kissing Games

Kissing is an incredibly intimate act that can be used to build anticipation and desire. Try playing a game where you take turns kissing each other in different ways, such as slow and sensual, or fast and playful. You might also try incorporating props like ice cubes or flavored lip gloss to add an extra element of excitement.

Sex in Public Places

While we certainly don't encourage breaking any laws, sex in public places can be an incredibly exciting and naughty experience. Consider exploring secluded areas like a park after hours or even your own backyard under the stars. Just remember to always be safe and respectful of others.

Incorporating Music and Lighting

Music and lighting are two elements that can help set the mood for a romantic and sensual night. Choose music that is sexy and sultry, and use dim lighting or candles to create a soft and warm atmosphere. You might even consider setting up a playlist beforehand that builds in intensity as your foreplay progresses. The right music and lighting can help create a sense of intimacy and passion, so don't overlook these important elements.

In conclusion, trying new tips and techniques in your foreplay routine can lead to greater sexual satisfaction and intimacy between partners. Whether it's exploring each other's erogenous zones, experimenting with temperature play, or incorporating food and drink, there are endless possibilities for spicing up your foreplay routine. Be open and communicate with each other, and don't be afraid to let your imagination run wild. Happy exploring!

V

Conclusion

Foreplay is an essential component of a fulfilling and satisfying sexual experience. By focusing on sensuality and intimacy, couples can create a deeper connection that enhances pleasure and mutual satisfaction. Throughout this book, we've explored a variety of tips and techniques that can be incorporated into your foreplay routine to heighten sensation and build anticipation.

While it may be tempting to stick with what you know, trying new things is key to keeping your sex life exciting and fulfilling. Don't be afraid to experiment with different types of touch, try new positions, or incorporate toys and props into your play. The possibilities for exploration are endless, so don't hesitate to get creative and adventurous.

However, it's important to remember that communication and consent should always be top priorities. Before trying any new techniques or ideas, make sure that both partners are on board and comfortable.

Some techniques, such as sensory deprivation or temperature play, may require more discussion and preparation than others. It's also important to establish boundaries and safe words beforehand to ensure that both partners feel secure and respected.

Above all, communication is essential to a successful and fulfilling sexual experience. Don't be afraid to talk to your partner about what feels good, what doesn't, and what you'd like to explore together. By prioritizing open and honest communication, you can build deeper trust and intimacy in your relationship.

In conclusion, incorporating foreplay into your sexual repertoire is key to maintaining a healthy and fulfilling sex life. Whether you're exploring new techniques, incorporating food and drink, or experimenting with sensory deprivation, there are endless possibilities for creating moments of intimacy and pleasure. Just remember to always prioritize communication and consent, and never be afraid to try something new. With these tools and techniques, you and your partner can take your foreplay routine to the next level and experience more profound and satisfying sexual experiences.

Thank you for taking the time to read this book and explore the world of foreplay together. By implementing these tips and techniques, you're sure to enhance your connection with your partner and create unforgettable moments of pleasure and intimacy. Remember to keep an open mind, listen to each other's desires and needs, and most importantly, have fun!

So go forth and explore the world of foreplay with renewed excitement and passion. You won't be disappointed!

www.ingramcontent.com/pod-product-compliance
Lightning Source LLC
Chambersburg PA
CBHW071554260726
48653CB00008BA/3173